SLEEPING HACKS

20+ Methods to Help You Sleep Better at Night

owners themselves, not affiliated with this document.

TABLE OF CONTENTS

INTRODUCTION

We all need sleep. Fact. Some people claim to thrive on just four hours a night, while others need over eight hours per night to exist. Whatever your personal preferences, we all know what it feels like to wake up tired after a restless night. Charging your internal batteries is essential and broken sleep patterns will lead to you feeling below par the day after.

This book is all about changing the way we prepare for bed, altering our habits and creating the perfect environment for sleep. Are you aware that your diet can help you sleep? Did you know that how you wake up is also important? Everything you need to know is here. Prepare yourself for the perfect sleep and wake up refreshed and invigorated.

CHAPTER 1: UNDERSTANDING THE FIVE STAGES OF SLEEP AND HOW WAKING UP IS JUST AS IMPORTANT

Are you aware that your sleep has different levels? Each level serves a different purpose. You will experience all five levels several times a night in a full night's sleep. If you wake in a certain stage of sleep, you can feel fully refreshed and yet a different stage will leave you wanting more despite sleeping for the same amount of time.

Before we get to the stages of the sleep cycle, it is important to identify the two types of sleep. REM and NREM stand for rapid eye movement and non-rapid eye movement. REM sleep is one of the five stages of the sleep cycle and occurs when we are dreaming. We could be in a fantasy world or just the normal world in which we live. We could be acting out moments of our past, or trying to create scenarios from our future.

Whatever and wherever we are our sleeping cycle are distinguished by the movement our eyes make under our closed eyelids. It would seem like our eyes are actually watching the dreams we are having and following the action. Hence the term rapid eye movement.

NREM sleep accounts for the remaining four patterns and can be described as the following:

- **Stage one:** This is the beginning of your sleep. The transition phase when you feel yourself drifting off and your breathing starts to slow. Stage one lasts up to ten minutes and sees the muscles relax and the heartbeat become regular. The eyes will roll back, and the eyelids can still be partially open. External stimuli or a simple touch from another person can cause a startling wake up for the sleeper.
If you allow yourself to wake naturally without the aid of an alarm you will wake up in stage one mode and feel refreshed.
- **Stage two:** This is another period of light sleep that lasts around twenty minutes. The heartbeat slows even further and the temperature of the body lowers. Brain activity begins to slow down as the body prepares to enter deeper sleep. It is more difficult to rouse someone from a stage two sleep than it is stage one.
- **Stage three:** This is when the body begins to enter a deep sleep, or delta sleep as it is also known. Stage three happens for around forty-five minutes and it is difficult to rouse someone from this stage. During stage three your brain waves slow to "delta waves" speed, but you can still experience short bursts of brain activity that are known as "beta waves." If you are woken from stage three sleep you will feel groggy and confused, unable to focus and slightly off-kilter.
- **Stage four:** This is the deepest stage of sleep and is the stage when your body restores itself, heals any injuries and encourages growth in adolescents. Your breathing will be rhythmic, and your brain will only produce delta waves during this cycle. While stage three will last for around fifteen minutes, stage four can last for up to an hour.
Children can experience bedwetting and night terrors during stage four sleep. Both adults and children can also sleep-

walk as they transcend from stage four sleep into a lighter stage.

Sleepwalking can run in the family and if you have a parent or sibling that sleepwalks you are ten times more likely to do so. Other causes of sleepwalking include:

- Stress
- Intoxication
- Sleep Deprived
- Drug-induced: particularly sedatives, stimulants, and antihistamines.

Certain medical problems can also cause the disorder

- Heart rhythm disorders
- Sleep apnea
- Restless leg syndrome
- Elevated body temperature due to fever
- Asthma
- Psychiatric disorders: Post-traumatic stress, panic attacks, and multiple personality disorders can all lead to sleepwalking.

Typically, a sleepwalker will just walk quietly around the room or they may run and attempt to escape. Sleepwalkers will also display open eyes and a fixed glassy stare and will normally be unresponsive. The best thing to do is to lead them back to bed without walking them.

- **Stage five:** This is the REM state and when we experience dreams. Studies have shown that dreaming is essential for our brain to sort through the countless pieces of information we collect during our waking hours. Some scientists believe that dreaming is a form of psychotherapy when we can address our unconscious desires and expectations.

During a sleep session, you may not experience all five stages of sleep. They are not sequential and can often be repeated during a sleep session. This explains why sometimes we can feel tired after a solid eight hours sleep yet feel refreshed after just five hours. The quality of sleep is determined by the sleep cycles you reach.

How to wake up properly!

Why is it that when the alarm goes off in the morning our instinct is to hit the snooze button? Even after a great night sleep we just want to pull the covers over our head and go back to sleep. Here are a few tips to help you change your attitudes to mornings:

- **Get excited about your day:** This is easy to do when it's a special day but what about a rainy Tuesday when you must go to work? Get creative and imagine all the great things that will happen during the day. Your first coffee, a chat with a friend or having lunch with your coworkers.
- **Natural light**: Once you are awake pull back the curtains and let the sunshine in! This is a natural way of telling your brain to start the day. Try waking up to a sunrise and drinking in the beauty of nature. This can be done from your bed but is so much better when you take a walk.
- **Drink water**: Often we wake up and start the day with a coffee. Consider the fact that your body will be slightly dehydrated as it hasn't had water for at least eight hours. Refresh your body with a long, cool glass of water before you reach for your cup of Joe.
- **Stretch**: Going from a prone position to an active one can cause problems for your joints. Have you ever watched cartoon characters get out of bed and stretch? This is actually a great way to get your circulation moving and help you feel more awake.

CHAPTER 2: HOW TO MAKE YOUR BEDROOM A RELAXING PLACE TO SLEEP

Ideally, your whole home should be a place that allows you to unwind. However, most of us know that there will always be the chaos of some sorts surrounding us. A noisy neighbor, a busy road or barking dogs can distract us and cause stress. Having a place to chill and relax is essential and as you drop off you should be in an environment that promotes relaxation.

Here are some great hacks to make your bedroom a haven of relaxation.

1) **Choose quality furniture:** When you are choosing the furniture for your bedroom pick quality pieces that are comfortable. When you go to a top-class hotel the first thing you notice is the bed and solid wood furniture. Surrounding yourself with craftsmanship will help you relax. Nobody wants to sleep surrounded by wobbly cheap furniture.

2) **Bedding:** When you have quality furniture you need to dress it with quality bedding. Choose pillows that will support your head properly, after all, you are going to spend eight hours a day lying on it! Consider how you sleep. If you sleep on your side, you will need a fuller pillow than if you sleep on your back.

Your sheets should be the softest, most luxurious you can afford. Thread count is the measure of threads per inch of bedding. The higher the count, the softer the sheet. Quality sheets will feel better on your skin and will also last longer.

3) **Regulate the temperature:** Your body temperature drops as you fall asleep. Having a cooler bedroom will help you fall asleep quicker as it jump-starts the cooling process. The ideal temperature is between 60 and 65 degrees.

4) **Mattress:** Do you find hotel beds comfier than your own? Chances are your mattress is letting you down. Sagging spots can affect your comfort and sleep quality. The natural life for a mattress is between eight and ten years and replacing it is important.

5) **Remove electronics:** Do you spend time in bed playing video games or watching TV? Maybe you need to check your social media before you drop off and whenever you wake during the night. Guess what, this is not good for you! Research has shown that removing all electronics from the bedroom can lead to an extra hour of sleep per night. This can be the difference between being tired the next morning and being fully refreshed.

6) **Alarm clock:** If you have removed all the electronics from your room how will you wake up? We all tend to use our smartphones as a wake-up call, but in reality, a traditional alarm clock is a lot better for our sleep quality. You can get digital models, but they will still glow in the dark. Why not go old school and use an old-fashioned wind-up alarm clock?

7) **Decorate your bedroom:** Color psychology is not an exact science, but there is a belief that you should choose colors that create a calming effect. If you want to avoid traditional beige and pastel shades, choose a color that creates an effect. Light purple contributes to restfulness while light brown creates a feeling of stability.

Don't be afraid of patterns, use rugs and throws to add color and interest to your room. Avoid neon colors and clashing patterns to create a feeling of calm.

A study by Travelodge showed that rooms painted blue, silver, yellow or green provided the most restful sleep for their customers.

8) **Aromatherapy**: Smells can help us relax and encourage sleep. Lavender and vanilla are effective and can also train our body to associate their smell with sleep. Using aromatherapy nightly will condition your body and mind to prepare for sleep.

If you use a diffuser and essential oils, you can become a master at creating the perfect scent to relax with. Here are a couple of blends that can aid you to sleep and relax you completely.

- Lavender, frankincense, and orange. The lavender is calming and relaxing for both physical and emotional balance. Frankincense has been used for thousands of years for medicinal purposes and lifts the spirits and enhances the mood. The orange essential oil will also add to the uplifting properties of the blend and promote relaxation.

- Lavender, lime, and chamomile: Lavender we know what to expect. The lime essential oil is known to support the respiratory system and chamomile helps combat depression.

9) **White noise:** A constant ambient sound will help eliminate loud noises and annoying background sounds. Anything that produces a constant sound can provide white noise, a fan or humidifier for instance. If you want to stay away from gadgets you can find a soundtrack to play on both Spotify and Pandora.

10) **Keep it clean:** Remove clutter and lessen stress levels. Your bedroom should have a bed, furniture, a few treasured pictures and accessories and nothing else. All shoes and clothes should be stored away. There should never be a desk or work area in your bedroom, you are there to relax! Now consider your bed. How great is it to snuggle up in clean sheets and

sweet-smelling bedding? Keep your bedding crisp and clean and improve your quality of sleep. When you get up in the morning make your bed before you leave for work. Studies showed that people who make their bed in the morning are 20% more likely to sleep well. Your bedroom is your haven, feeling good about it can only help the sleeping process.

Final tip: Sleep and intimacy are the only two purposes your bedroom should have! No work, no TV or gaming, just sleep, and sex! Condition your mind to accept this and you will learn to love your special room and how it makes you feel.

CHAPTER 3: WHAT YOU SHOULD AND SHOULDN'T WEAR TO BED

We know that sleep is intrinsically linked to our health and how important our surroundings are. Have you considered your bedtime attire choices and how they can impact on the quality of your sleep? Are you putting yourself at risk of serious health problems just by putting your pajamas on?

Here are some tips to help you wear the right nighttime attire

1) **Ditch the underwear**
   Wearing underwear to bed is a practice that is common especially for women. However, consider the following facts before you wear your pants and bra to bed! Wearing underwear creates the perfect breeding ground for bacteria. Moist dark and warm areas encourage the development of vaginal and yeast infections.
   Wearing a bra to bed is also thought to prevent sagging in the future, but this is a common misconception. If the bra is tight fitting you can hinder your circulation and put unnecessary pressure on your chest. The hooks, under wires, and straps of the bra can also cause irritating welts, indentations and even cysts. Wearing a bra to bed also increases the likelihood of developing an infection if your bedroom is

warm.

Going commando to bed will feel unusual at first, but it is worth persevering. The ease and simplicity will help you sleep better ad it can also increase intimacy levels with your partner. Need another reason for ditching your underwear? How about less laundry? So, less chance of infection, more intimacy, and less laundry result!

2) **Keep it loose**

We are all aware of the ranges of tight fitting and flattering nightwear that women can wear to bed and how it can make us feel sexy and attractive. The truth is that these types of nightwear should be restricted to special occasions as they are restricting the ability for your body to breathe naturally and hampering your circulation.

Replace the booty shorts and spandex negligees with cotton vests and loose fitting sweat pants or cotton shorts. Loose fitting cotton pajamas may not raise the temperature of your partner, but they will help you regulate your own. If you tend to overheat during the night cotton will help you cool down. If you tend to feel chilly when sleeping a thicker material may suit you better. Classic flannel fabric pajamas can offer you a better option, especially during winter and fall.

If you are looking for an option that is both sexy and beneficial to your health what about silk? Ultra-luxurious and a perfect way to regulate your body's temperature it may be worth investing in a super sexy pair of silk pajamas.

3) **Keep it clean**

Once you have your favorite nightwear there is a tendency to wear it every night and fail to wash it sufficiently. The average person loses millions of skin cells and up to a quart of sweat daily chances are your pajamas are not as clean as you think! They need to be washed after wearing them three times, but that may not be convenient for everyone. Consider having multiple pairs of your favorite jammies and avoid wearing dirty pajamas.

4) **Keep your feet warm**

Cold feet are a common reason for lack of sleep, but there is a physical reason for this. Warming up your feet helps lower your blood pressure that is a natural way to prepare your body for sleep. Studies have shown that warm feet will help you fall asleep faster. Did you know that socks can be a beauty aid for your feet? Wearing them in bed helps prevent dryness and cracked heels and helps you keep your feet looking youthful and beautiful.

You can also use socks to absorb moisture if your feet are on the sweaty side and avoid placing your sweaty feet on your partner. Choose comfortable cotton socks, which have loose elastic, and make them a part of your nighttime routine.

5) **Ditch the jewelry**

Do you regularly go to bed in your favorite earrings and necklace? Have you always slept with your engagement and wedding rings on? Maybe the thought of removing these special and significant items has never entered your head. Wearing jewelry can be disastrous in bed and you could be exposing yourself to skin irritations and allergic reactions.

How many times have you woken up with indentations or scratches from your jewelry? Have you ever caught your hair in your jewelry or snagged yourself on the bedding? The potential for choking or causing circulation issues are vastly increased when you go to bed in your jewelry. You may love your bling but removing your precious items will help you sleep safer.

6) **Hair care**

Wearing something on your head may seem somewhat unusual but consider how your hair is damaged during sleep. Rubbing your head against a pillow for eight hours can lead to frizz and hair breakage. Wearing a silk scarf to bed will keep your hair from drying out and give you a silky, smooth mane to be proud of. Covering long hair will also cut down on tangles and split ends.

7) **Cover up**

External factors can hinder your ability to sleep and unless you live in an area that has no noise disturbances you will come across these factors. A noisy neighbor, a howling dog or external lights can disturb you and create annoying distractions. Closer to home a snoring partner can keep you awake all night so what can you do to block these distractions?

Earplugs and a sleep mask will help you eliminate these external factors and improve your sleep. Having your eyes and ears covered in bed may feel unusual at first, but the benefits are worth it. Studies have shown that wearing a sleep mask and earplugs will also raise natural levels of melatonin that promotes healthy sleep.

Sleeping nude with a pair of socks, an eye mask, and earplugs seem to be the perfect way to get a decent night's sleep. Place your jewelry on your nightstand and put your silk scarf on and you are good to go! Of course, not everyone will embrace all the tips we have mentioned, but you should be able to benefit from at least one or two of them.

CHAPTER 4: NATURAL WAYS TO AID SLEEP

Meditation and relaxation techniques

Your stress levels can affect your sleep and it can be difficult to lower them. Using meditation and other relaxation techniques can slow your breathing and direct your attention to an object of focus. When your mind is filled with outside stimuli it can be hard to relax. These techniques will help you concentrate and increase awareness.

- **Visualization:** Involve all your senses and imagine a place that relaxes you. Think of a beach with the sea lapping at the shores and the feel of sunshine on your bare skin. You can hear the waves, smell the sea and feel the warm breeze on your skin. Imagine lying back on a towel and closing your eyes. Drift off to the sound of the ocean and the warmth of the summer sun.
- **Mindfulness**: Focus on the positive aspects of your life and what you can do to improve them. Appreciate all the great connections you have with your family and friend and thank the universe for the joy in your life.
- **7-11 breathing technique**: This technique is designed to regulate your breathing and prepare you for sleep. Breathe in for 7 seconds and then breathe out for 11 seconds. Lay in your favorite position and repeat until you fall asleep. The constant counting will help you focus on your mind, muscles, and body and help them relax.

- **Squeeze and relax:** As you are lying in bed focus on one group of muscles at a time. Squeeze them until tense and then relax them. Your mind will be calmed by the actions and your body will relax.

Herbal Sleep Aids

The herb Vitex Agnus Castus - also known as chaste tree - can help cure insomnia during menstruation. Studies have shown that women suffering from PMS can benefit from taking the chaste tree. However, this herb should not be taken when on birth control pills, hormone replacement therapy or any dopamine-based medication.

Valerian is an herbal home-brewed remedy that can provide relief from insomnia and aid sleep. A standard dose of 450mg should be taken an hour before bedtime and should be taken with food. Valerian is thought to increase the levels of calming neutron transmitters in the body and can relieve muscle spasms.

Lemon balm is available as a supplement or in tea form and is said to relieve anxiety and calm the nervous system. Sleep aid supplements with lemon balm generally contain valerian as well.

General hacks for a better sleep

- No pets: This can be a tough one for some people, but you can't expect a good night's sleep when you have your fluffy companions in your bed. Studies have shown that you are 63% more likely to have a poor night's sleep if your pets are with you.
- Sleep on the left side of your body: Experts recommend sleeping on your left as it improves your circulation and combats heartburn and acid reflux. You are also less likely to be interrupted.
- Don't look at the clock: Sneaking a peek at the clock to see how long it is before you wake up will only cause you anxiety.
- Don't leave things undone: Doing the washing up and other

unpleasant tasks before you go to bed will help you relax. If you are worried about paying the bills or general household tasks you will be less likely to relax.

- Take a cold bath: We all know the benefits of a warm bath but can a cold dip before bedtime do you good? Experts have proved that a cold bath an hour before sleep can help lower the temperatures of the body. This helps the process of falling to sleep and is like being hit with a tranquilizer.

- Allow your feet freedom: When you are dreaming or having a nightmare you will often imagine running or moving your feet. If your bedclothes are restricting your feet you will feel anxious and this can wake you up even when you are experiencing deep sleep.

Have you considered the position you sleep in? There are studies that show instinctive sleeping patterns that nomads and forest dwellers adapt can help with musculoskeletal health and help correct joint pain.

Mountain gorillas naturally sleep on one side and use a laterally rotated arm as a pillow. Native Kenyans adopt the same position that allows them to listen for danger with both ears.

Tibetan caravanners have been pictured sleeping on their shins. This position may seem unnatural for the "civilized" world, but nature tells us differently. The anterior border of the tibia and the medial border of the ulna are the only parts of the body that are in contact with the ground when sleeping in this position. This minimizes the loss of heat while the folded position of the body also conserves heat. The position also allows the sleeper to have both ears alert for any foe and prevents them from revealing their position by making a noise. As the head is facing down this closes the mouth and makes it impossible to snore.

Of course, we are not suggesting you abandon your pillows and sleep like a gorilla or indeed a Tibetan caravanner, but a change of position might make all the difference. Try sleeping in the military crawl position and limit the movement of your body during sleep. Lie face down on your bed and tilt your head to expose your right cheek. Lift your right arm into a crooked position so it points above your head. Your right leg should be bent at the knee and face outward at an angle to your stomach.

Imagine a soldier crawling under a net and replicate the position. Some cultures use this position to prevent babies and younger children from moving when they need to be calm. Less movement means faster sleep.

Final note: Some people are just not meant to sleep in the same bed. We may love the idea of spooning with our partners until we both drift off into a romantic sleep and waking in a mutual embrace. The reality is that your partner may snore, pass wind or just take all the bedding. If you find you are losing sleep because of your partner, consider sleeping in different beds. Different schedules and even different temperature preferences can cause a loss of sleep. You may even find yourself enjoying the time you do spend together in the bedroom more knowing that you are going to sleep well after! Remember the two things the bedroom is for? Why not improve both?

CHAPTER 5: HOW DOES YOUR DIET AFFECT YOUR SLEEP?

We need to know what our body does to induce sleep before we examine what the best foods are for a successful sleep cycle. There are four main minerals that aid sleeping. Tryptophan, Magnesium, Calcium, and B6. It is possible to ingest these minerals in supplements, but the best way is to add them to your diet.

Here are the best foods to add to your diet for each of the main minerals

1) **Tryptophan:** This is an amino acid that encourages your pineal gland to produce melatonin. As your natural bedtime approaches your body will automatically release melatonin into your bloodstream and help you prepare for sleep.
   - Organic meats: Lamb, beef, liver, chicken, pork, venison.
   - Seafood: Mackerel, tuna, shrimp, halibut, herring, crab, lobster.
   - Dairy products: Yogurt, cheese, milk, cream.
   - Fresh fruit: Avocados, cherries, mango, pineapple, oranges, mandarins, bananas, kiwi.
   - Fresh vegetables: All green vegetables, spinach, parsnips, mushrooms.
   - Nuts: Small amounts of high-fat nuts such as peanuts, almonds, and cashews.

- Whole grains: Bulgur, barley, red rice, corn, oats.
- Legumes: Chickpeas, cannellini beans, fava beans, French green beans, lentils, lima bean, runner bean, sugar snap pea.

2) **Magnesium:** This natural sedative helps your body relax as it controls your adrenaline levels. Your hydration levels are improved with a healthy level of magnesium and your muscles find it easier to relax. Here are the foods that will help you boost your levels:
- Fish: Salmon, cod, herring, mackerel.
- Legumes: Small red bean, kidney bean, frijol bola roja, green and yellow peas, alfalfa.
- Dark leafy vegetables: Kale, mustard greens, cabbage, broccoli, arugula, chard, collard greens.
- Bananas
- Low-fat dairy products: Goat cheese, cottage cheese, yogurt.
- Grains
- Dried fruits: Raisins, cranberries, dates, pineapple, apricots.

3) **Calcium:** We are all aware of the need for calcium to help strengthen teeth and bones, but did you know it can also help you sleep? Calcium will help your brain process tryptophan to produce melatonin that aids sleep. It also regulates blood pressure and improves muscle contraction and expansion.
These calcium-rich foods will help prevent insomnia:
- Chinese cabbage: Bok choy, Pak Choy.
- Soy products: Tofu, soybean, soymilk.
- Okra
- Cruciferous leafy greens
- Edible green leaves: Dandelion, red clover, watercress, chickweed, plantain.
- Oily fish; Anchovies, herring, tuna, salmon.

4) **B6:** Your body needs serotonin. This is a neurotransmitter that promotes sleep and regulates sleep cycles. Vitamin B6 helps the brain to convert a small amount of tryptophan into serotonin. These foods will help you keep you maintain a healthy level of B6 in your diet:

- Organic meat: Steak, beef, venison, chicken, pork, mutton, lamb.
- Seafood: Swordfish, lobster, cod, halibut, mussels, salmon.
- Dried fruits
- Avocados
- Cruciferous leafy greens: Kale, mustard green, cabbage, broccoli.
- Chickpeas
- Garlic
- Tuna
- Spinach

What drinks can help you achieve a better sleep pattern?

Minerals are not only found in food but also in beverages. A nighttime drink can fit perfectly into your bedtime routine and boost your mineral levels. Drinking one of the following drinks before you go to bed will condition your body to prepare for sleep as well as boosting your mineral levels.

- **Warm milk**: Filled with calcium and tryptophan; this is the perfect way to trigger the body's natural "sleepy" hormone, melatonin.
- **Cocoa:** If warm milk doesn't float your boat try cocoa. The Mayans were one of the first people to drink cocoa and prepared it with roasted cocoa beans, hot water, and spices.
- **Chamomile tea:** The lack of caffeine and the gentle flavor means that chamomile is great for relaxing the mind and body. It calms the nerves and settles the stomach making it a perfect way to prepare for bed.

- **Passionfruit tea:** Another delicate drink that soothes the nerves, passionfruit tea is packed with healthy minerals.
- **Valerian tea:** Made from essential oils obtained from the roots of the valerian plant this herbal tea promotes healthy sleep and can also decrease stress. This tea is especially effective for women with menstrual problems.
- **Tart cherry juice:** This is the best source of natural melatonin.

If you want to sweeten any of the above drinks use honey instead of refined sugar and add a healthy dose of natural sweetener.

Food and drinks to avoid

- **Alcohol:** Many people believe a nightcap will help them sleep, but in reality, it will interfere with your sleep cycles.
- **Caffeine:** Avoid all caffeine after 2 pm to help you aid sleep. There are some surprising sources of caffeine, here are some products you may not realize contain caffeine: Energy water, pain relievers, regular and diet sodas, chocolate, and decaf coffees. Decaf products are not necessarily caffeine free, check the levels of all these products.
- **Fast food:** All fast food will take longer to digest than healthy snacks. If food is lying in your stomach it will prevent you from relaxing properly.
- **High-fat foods**
- **Spicy foods**
- **Refined carbs**: Bread, white rice, cakes, cookies, crackers, pie, and candy.
- **Pasta**
- **Nicotine**

If you need a snack before bedtime, there are a couple of great recipes that are healthy and will not interrupt your sleep. Try these healthy evening snacks for a feel-good factor before bedtime.

Banana peanut bagel

The tryptophan-rich bananas combined with magnesium packed peanut butter will help relax the muscles and work as a mild relaxant to the nervous system.

Ingredients

1 overripe banana

½ whole meal bagel

1 Tbsp natural crunchy peanut butter

Mash the banana in a bowl. Toast the bagel and spread it with peanut butter. Top with the mashed banana and serve.

Green fruit salad

Makes 4 servings

Ingredients

2 cups of honeydew melon

½ cup of seedless grapes

½ cup peeled ripe kiwi fruit cut into quarters

A ½ cup of yogurt

A squirt of lime juice

2 tbsp fresh mint

Combine the fruit and refrigerate up to 4 hours before serving. Serve with yogurt and lime juice and top with fresh mint.

Almond butter and banana smoothie

Ingredients

1 small frozen banana

1 cup almond milk

1 tbsp honey

½ tsp ground cinnamon

Combine all the ingredients in a blender and mix until smooth, Ice cubes can be added to cool the smoothie if required.

As with any food these foods are best eaten at least an hour before bedtime.

CHAPTER 6: SLEEP DESTROYING HABITS AND HOW TO BREAK THEM

Sleep quality is essential. Humans spend one-third of their lives sleeping. Consider how you plug your electronic devices into the mains to recharge. Sleep s your charger and it helps you regenerate and recharge your batteries.

These are the most common reasons that our sleep patterns are disrupted:

- **Stress**
  In our busy world stress is the number one killer of the 21st century. We are all guilty of lying in our bed worrying about work, relationships and other factors in our lives. Clearing your mind may seem impossible, but it is essential that you go to bed with a stress-free mind. Watch a humorous clip online or read a funny quote. Does a particular activity always make you smile? Make sure you do it before you go to bed. Your state of mind should be optimistic and carefree. Worrying about cash or work will not solve anything, it will only leave you tired and irritable in the morning.
- **Poor mental activity**
  Intense light prevents the body from producing melatonin and stimulates the mind. Switch off the TV or computer

screen and practice a restorative action instead. Read a book using an incandescent lamp or take a gentle walk in the garden. Practice yoga or meditation before bedtime and feel the benefit of a calm mind and a relaxed body.

- **Room temperature**
This is a personal choice should be tailored to the individual. People have an internal physical clock that regulates your core temperature. Your body needs to be cool when sleeping as heat tells your inner clock that it is time to get up. If your body warms up in the middle of the night you will automatically wake. There is no optimum temperature that works for everyone as we all have different metabolisms. Make sure your room is at the right temperature for you and feel the benefits while you sleep.

- **Supplements and medication**
We have already discussed the caffeine in some pain restrictors, but there are other drugs that can affect your sleep. Steroids and beta-blockers can contain stimulants and affect your sleep and keep you awake at night. Vitamin B supplements should be taken before 2 p.m. to avoid it disrupting your sleep. Whenever you are prescribed new medications or are considering additional supplements, ask your doctor or pharmacist to make sure your sleep will not be affected.

- **Exposure to artificial light**
How often have you been on your computer or smartphone just before bedtime and all you can see when you close your eyes is a screen? You need to prioritize your sleep and shun the devices. Artificial lights combined with the poor mental activity we have already mentioned are key factors to sleep deprivation.

- **Eating too much food**
When you have a busy schedule, it can be tempting to eat a huge meal once you get home and then go to bed. Socializing can also involve eating later than normal and going to sleep with a full stomach. Heartburn and lack of digestion

will disturb your sleeping patterns and keep you awake.

Sometimes we need to sleep even when we are not tired. If you follow the tips that we have covered but are still wide awake what can you do to fall asleep?

- **Play soothing music:** Create a playlist with songs that have a slow rhythm (60 to 80 beats a minute) and listen for 30 minutes before falling to sleep. There is a list of suitable songs on Spotify named the 20 most streamed tracks for sleep. Avoid ear buds or headphones and invest in pillow speakers.

- **Breathe only through your left nostril:** Are you aware that during the day you alternate your breathing between your left and right nostril? When you breathe through your right nostril you are more alert and when you breathe through your left nostril you feel relaxed and calmer. Induce sleep and relaxation by actively breathing through your left nostril using the following techniques:
    - Block your right nostril with your right thumb
    - Take long, steady breaths through your left nostril
    - Repeat and continue for up to 10 minutes until it feels like you are dominantly using your left nostril
    - Sleep on your right side to help your left nostril breathe freely

- **Dipping your face in cold water:** We have already discovered that a lower body temperature helps induce sleep. If you are wide awake, try filling a sink with cold water and some cold packs from the freezer. Immerse your face for 30 seconds and this will make your blood pressure and heart rate to drop. This technique is known as Cold Thermogenesis and is a tried and tested way to sleep when not tired.

- **Use Acupressure:** The therapy of acupressure involves the placing of fingers with levels of pressure on specific points of the body. Normally a massage therapist would administer acupressure, but this simple method can be self-administered using the following method:

- Locate the acupressure point known as the Inner Gate. This is the central point of the inner side of the forearm, two and a half fingers from the crease at your wrist.
- Stimulate the point by placing the right thumb on the inner side of your left wrist and apply pressure for 90 seconds. Change position by applying pressure to the same point on the opposite arm for 90 seconds. Repeat until you feel relaxed.

There are many different points to use acupressure depending on the result you wish to achieve. Natural methods like acupressure and reflexology help us to achieve improved sleep without resorting to medicinal aids.

These hacks will all benefit your sleep and when combined with a healthy diet and exercise routine will enhance your overall well-being. If you suffer from insomnia you will feel sluggish, melancholy and can also be lacking in focus. Your health can suffer, and you risk suffering from diabetes, cancer, coronary illness, and diminished libido.

CONCLUSION

You now have the hacks you need to get a full night's sleep and face the world with added energy. Enjoy your mornings and keep away from that snooze button!

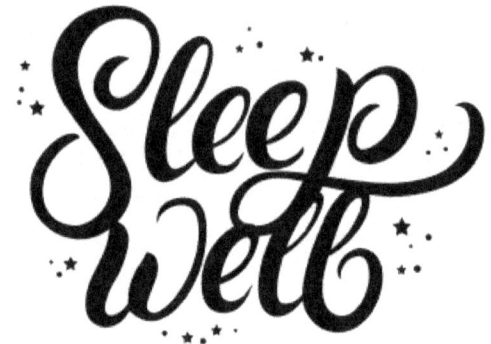

And finally, if you liked the book, I would like to ask you to do me a favor and leave a review for the book on Amazon.

Thank you and good luck!